Coconut Oil

The Best 25 Ways On How To Use Coconut Oil For Beauty, Hair, Health, Increasing Energy, and Losing Weight

Table of Contents

Introduction

Chapter One – Why Coconut Oil Can Help You Increase Your Energy Levels

Chapter Two – How Coconut Oil Can Help You Lose Weight

Chapter Three – The Top Ways Coconut Oil Nourishes All Hair Types

Chapter Four – Unexpected Beauty Uses for Coconut Oil

Chapter Five - Using Coconut Oil as an Alternate Treatment for Illnesses and Disease

Chapter Six – Coconut Oil for the Home

Chapter Seven – Finding the Right Coconut Oil for Your Needs

Conclusion

FREE BONUSES

Introduction

More than ninety percent of coconut oil is saturated fats, along with traces of a few unsaturated fatty acids, like polyunsaturated fatty acids and monounsaturated fatty acids. Virgin coconut oil is no different. However, it's not bad for your heart at all! In fact, coconut oil has been proven to be healthy for your heart.

The saturated fats in coconut oil are mostly medium chain fatty acids, which agree with the body's systems well. Lauric acid is the chief medium chain fatty acid found in coconut oil, and represents more than forty percent of the total, followed up by capric acid, caprylic acid, palmitic, and myristic acid. The body creates monolaurin from lauric acid, which is helpful in handling diseases and viruses. The capric acid reacts with enzymes that are created by bacteria. It's then converted into an antimicrobial known as monocaprin. Caproic, caprylic, and myristic acid are also antimicrobial and antifungal in nature.

The unsaturated fatty acids are polyunsaturated fatty acids and monounsaturated fatty acids. Coconut oil also has Gallic acid, which is also called phenolic acid. It also contains many different vitamins and nutrients that are important for your overall health.

The point is this. Coconut oil is very healthy for you and can be used as an antifungal, antibacterial, and antiviral. It helps with weight loss, digestive upset, and many other illnesses, as well as substitutes for beauty and hair treatment, and is great as an alternative, organic cleaner!

You can find out more about all its beneficial uses in this book, as well as a comprehensive guide on which coconut oils will suit your needs best.

Chapter One – Why Coconut Oil Can Help You Increase Your Energy Levels

Consuming coconut oil boosts your energy level like premium grade gasoline boosts the performance of a sports car. The metabolism in the body shifts into a higher gear when coconut oil is consumed.

Many of us lack energy and are easily fatigued, but coconut oil can help alleviate this problem. Many people automatically believe this translates to coconut oil being like caffeine, but it's more subtle than that and it lasts much longer than the short boost a cup of coffee gives you. Unlike a cup of coffee, the effects of coconut oil last for hours and you don't develop an addiction or dependence on it like you would coffee.

You may have heard about the medium chain fatty acids and how they have an effect on your metabolism and energy, but most people don't connect coconut oil with this type of fatty acid. In reality, coconut oil is basically nothing but medium chain fatty acids! That's why you should never take it before bed. You'll be up all night thinking about all the things you should be doing rather than sleeping!

Rather than drinking coffee in the morning to wake up for just an hour, a little coconut oil will do the same thing to help you through the morning routine or that afternoon slump without the terrible side effect of crashing an hour later. A tablespoon of coconut oil in a cup of herbal tea or some juice will boost your energy.

The effects of medium-chain fatty acids in coconut oil are so great that researchers are investigating their use for enhancing athletic performance and endurance. Results of these studies are encouraging, yet they're mild when compared to drugs. In Australia, horse trainers feed the horses a coconut cake that has about ten percent coconut oil because it enhances their performance.

Medium chain fatty acid oils are added to sports drinks and energy drinks in order to give athletes a boost. Even if you're not an athlete, you can still enjoy the benefits of coconut oil.

Coconut oil works best if it's consumed half an hour before you plan on doing any type of exercise work as it takes a bit to take effect.

Chapter Two – How Coconut Oil Can Help You Lose Weight

If coconut oil gives you energy and boosts your metabolism, then it can help you lose weight, right? Coconut oil is very different from any other fats in our diet. Where most foods have long-chain fatty acids, coconut oil is mostly medium-chain. Medium-chained fatty acids are metabolized differently than any other type of fatty acid by going straight to the liver from our digestive tracts. This is where they're used for energy immediately or turned into ketone bodies.

These fats are usually used be epileptic patients on a ketogenic diet to increase their ketone levels and allow for more carbohydrates in their diet at the same time. There's also evidence from animal studies that the medium chain fats are stored less efficiently than others. In one study conducted with rats, they were fed medium chain fats and gained twenty percent less weight, as well as twenty-three percent less body fat.

The bottom line is that coconut oil helps you burn fat rather than gain it!

A Calorie Is Not a Calorie

Calories are not all the same. Different macronutrients and foods go through different metabolic pathways in the body. The different types of food you eat have an effect on your metabolic health and your hormones. Some metabolic pathways are more efficient and some foods require more energy in order to digest and metabolize.

One property about coconut oil is that it's thermogenic, meaning consuming it tends to increase your energy expenditure compared to the same amount of calories from any other fat. In one study, one to two tablespoons were shown to increase energy expenditure by five percent, which totaled around 120 calories a day.

Several others confirmed these findings. When humans replace the fats they consume with coconut oil or medium chain fatty acids, they are burning more calories. Therefore, a calorie from coconut oil is not the same as a calorie from olive oil or butter.

Reduces Appetite

Weight loss is about calories coming in and calories going out. Even though this is a little bit of a drastic simplification, it is true. If your body uses more calories than it consumes, then you'll lose fat. But even though it's true we have to be calorie deficient in order to lose weight, it doesn't mean calories or something you need to count or consciously be aware of.

Humans are capable of being healthy and lean in a natural environment. The obesity epidemic did not occur until the 1980's, and we didn't know what a calorie was a hundred years ago. Anything that reduces your appetite makes you take in fewer calories without having to think about it. It appears coconut oil has that effect.

Numerous studies have shown that compared to the same amount of calories that come from other fats, coconut oil increases the feelings of fullness and leads to an automatic reduction in calories consumed. This might be related to the way the fats are processed. It's well known that ketone bodies have an appetite reducing effect, and coconut oil is turned into this in the liver.

In one study conducted with six healthy men, eating a high amount of medium-chain fatty acids caused them to eat 256 fewer calories a day. In another study with fourteen healthy men, those who consumed medium chain fatty acids at breakfast ate a lot fewer calories at lunch. Therefore, coconut oil boosts your fat burning capabilities and it reduces your appetite.

Helps You Lose Unsafe Abdominal Fat

If coconut oil is able to boost your metabolic rate and decrease your appetite, then it's able to help you lose weight long[-term. There are many studies that support this theory. In one study, forty women were given two tablespoons of coconut oil or soybean oil for twenty-eight days. They were instructed to eat fewer calories every day and walk. Both groups lost about two pounds. Only the coconut oil decreased their belly fat while the soybean oil participants had an increase in belly fat. The coconut oil group had reduced the HDL cholesterol levels while the soybean oil reduced HDL and increased LDL, the bad cholesterol.

In this study, coconut oil didn't cause overall weight loss compared to the soybean oil, but it did lead to a significant reduction in abdominal fat. In another study with obese men, thirty grams of coconut oil were given daily for four weeks, which reduced the men's waists by 1.1 inches. There are also studies that have shown medium chain fats lead to weight loss, reduced waist size, and improvements in metabolic health.

While the weight loss effects of coconut oil are mild when it's the only source used, its effects on abdominal fat are phenomenal. Visceral fat is the fat that builds up around the organs and can cause cardiovascular disease, inflammation, and diabetes. Any reduction in abdominal fat will have a positive effect on your metabolic health and reduce your risk of chronic disease.

These results may not be shocking or dramatic, but consider that all these people did was add coconut oil to their diet. Combined with other ways to lose weight, such as increasing your protein intake and cutting out carbohydrates, this can lead to a significant amount of weight lost.

Therefore, coconut oil supports a healthy, read-food based weight loss diet.

Calories in Coconut Oil

It is imperative you keep in mind that coconut oil is fat. Fat has nine calories for every gram, and coconut oil is not an exception to this rule. Therefore, if you eat a fixed amount of calories every day and you add the coconut oil on top of that, then you will gain weight and not lose weight. However, most people are not counting calories and eating a fixed amount every day.

In this case, adding coconut oil to your diet can reduce your appetite and make you eat less of the other foods instead. So it's not really about adding fat calories to the diet, but about replacing some of the other fats you consume with the coconut oil.

It's also important to note that you shouldn't add tons of coconut oil to your diet and go overboard. The studies you read about used two tablespoons per day of oil. As we all know, consuming too much oil can cause some gastrointestinal upset, and in this case, more is not always better.

But coconut oil is not only great for weight loss! It's also good for nourishing any type of hair. Read about that in the next chapter.

Chapter Three – The Top Ways Coconut Oil Nourishes All Hair Types

There are so many reasons coconut oil is excellent for any hair type out there. First and foremost, it keeps your hair hydrated without causing a greasy residue, which is excellent for hair types that have greasy hair! Read about why in this chapter.

Deep Conditioning

Due to coconut oil being mainly made of smaller MCT's, the oil of the coconut will penetrate the hair shaft faster than any other conditioner. To use it as a leave-in treatment to repair split ends, simply moisturize the scalp and add a healthy glow by following these steps:

1. Be sure you have an hour or two for this treatment. The longer you leave the coconut oil in the hair, the more effective it will be.

2. Wash your hair and allow it to air dry as you prepare the following steps.

3. Gather the materials. You'll need a hair pick or comb, a shower cap, a small

towel to wrap around your head, two small bowls with one that fits into the other, and your jar of organic coconut oil.

4. Scoop a small amount of the oil into the smaller bowl.

5. Set the smaller in the bottom of the larger bowl.

6. Fill the bigger bowl with warm water and let the smaller bowl sit in it without floating.

7. Once the oil is to temperature and has melted, use your fingers to massage it into your hair and then work it through with a comb or a hair pick.

8. After you're done applying it, wrap your hair in a shower cap or a small towel and let it soak for half an hour or longer.

9. Shampoo your hair to remove the excess oil.

10. You can also reapply a small amount of the oil to the ends of your hair again if it needs a healthy shine.

You can then just style as usual after you're finished! Your hair will be soft, shiny, and your split ends will be mended.

Daily Detangler

Anyone who has long or curly hair knows that dealing with tangles is a daily battle. Coconut oil helps with this, too. Due to it being a natural oil, you won't leave any residue or long-term damage in your hair. Before you brush or style your hair, follows these steps to use coconut oil as a detangler.

1. Gather your tools. You'll need a hair brush, comb, or a pick, two small bowls that are of different sizes, and your coconut oil.

2. Take a bit of the oil and add it to the smaller of the two bowls and set the smaller one inside the larger one. Put a little warm water in the larger one and wait for the oil to melt.

3. Use your fingers to gently add the oil to the ends of our hair, and then begin from the ends and work your up toward the roots gently.

4. Let the oil soak in, and then brush and style it as usual. There's no need to rinse or shampoo, allowing the oil to nourish your hair all day.

Defeat Dandruff

If you have used chemical shampoos, styling products, conditioners, and colorants for a long time, you've most likely developed a flaky and itchy scalp. This is dandruff, and you can use coconut oil to nourish your hair and heal your scalp. Just follow these easy steps every day and your dandruff will disappear!

1. And the end of the day, right before you go to bed, wash your hair with a natural shampoo and condition it as you usually do.

2. Gather up a comb, two small bowls of different sizes, a towel or cap to cover your hair overnight, and a jar of coconut oil.

3. Scoop a bit of the oil into the small of the two bowls and put it in the bottom of the larger one.

4. Put hot water in the larger bowl and wait for the oil to melt in the smaller one.

5. As you wait for the oil to get to room temperature, remove any tangles from your hair.

6. Once the oil has melted, use your fingers to massage the oil into your scalp gently. If you have long hair, it might be easier to flip your head down so that you can apply the oil to your entire scalp.

7. Wrap your head with the towel or a cap and leave the oil on your scalp overnight for the best results.

8. The next morning, use an Epsom salt treatment to remove the excess skin cells on your scalp.

Base for Hair Coloring

Coconut oil is an excellent medium for mixing with an all-natural hair coloring. Due to coconut oil penetrating the hair deeper and faster than most other natural oils, it helps the color be more vibrant and stops it from fading right away.

1. Gather the materials. You need a small towel or shower cap, a hair pick, coloring herbs, two bowls of different sizes, gloves, a container for mixing the color, and the jar of organic coconut oil.

2. Scoop a few tablespoons of the oil into the smaller of the two bowls and set it in the bottom of the larger bowl. Put warm water in the larger bowl and wait for the oil to melt. It should be enough oil to liberally coat your hair.

3. Mix the oil with the coloring herbs and apply it as you normally would. Once the color has set, shampoo your hair with lukewarm water to remove any excess oil and colorant.

4. Wrap your hair with a shower cap or a towel and allow the color to set overnight.

Faster Hair Growth

Coconut oil is an excellent way to make your hair grow thicker, long, and fuller faster. The vitamins and the MCT's in the coconut oil nourish your scalp and help to remove the sebum build-up from your hair follicles. Use coconut oil as a daily treatment like this.

1. At the end of the day or just before bedtime, wash your hair with your natural shampoo and condition it as you usually do.

2. Gather the materials. You'll need a comb, a shower cap, two small bowls of different sizes, and a jar of coconut oil.

3. Scoop some of the oil into the smaller of the two bowls and set the smaller one in the larger one. Pour some warm water into the larger one and wait for the oil to melt.

4. While you wait for the oil to melt, use the comb or the pick to remove any tangles.

5. Once the oil has fully melted, use your fingers to fully massage it into the scalp. If you have long hair, flip your head down so you can reach the scalp better.

6. Wrap your head with a towel or use the shower cap and let it soak overnight for the best results.

Protect Hair from Sun Damage

Coconut oil is a natural sunscreen. In the morning, especially on days when you know your hair is going to be exposed to the elements more than it usually is, apply the oil to protect your hair by using these steps.

1. Gather your materials. You'll need a comb, two small bowls of differing sizes, and the coconut oil.

2. Scoop a small amount of oil into the smaller of the two bowls and put warm water in the larger one. Wait for the oil to fully melt.

3. Use your fingers to massage the oil into your hair and then brush and style it as you usually would.

For Greasy Hair

If you're someone who suffers from greasy hair, you know how difficult it is to get rid of it without making the rest of your hair dry and brittle in the process. Most of the time, greasy hair comes from stripping out too much of the natural sebum or oils in the hair as we're shampooing. Use coconut oil as a conditioner after you shower and allow it to stay in your hair all day long. It will keep your hair from getting greasy because the coconut oil helps keep sebum from building up!

But coconut oil is not only for your hair! It can be used on any part of your body for beauty purposes. Read about how in the following chapter.

Chapter Four – Surprising Beauty Usages for Coconut Oil

Coconut oil is an excellent way to simplify your beauty routine! You can use it on just about any part of the body. Take a look at these ideas for your next beauty routine.

Makeup Remover

Even the most waterproof mascara and lipstick doesn't stand a chance when it comes to coconut oil. Apply is directly to your face as an oil cleanser or allow it to sit on your skin with a cotton pad. The makeup will literally wipe right off! An added benefit is that it cleanses and softens your skin at the same time.

Breath Freshener

Coconut oil is a natural antibacterial and antifungal, so gargling with it for twenty minutes helps clear up germs in your mouth. This leads to fresher breath, healthier gums, and whiter teeth. It's known as oil pulling because the oil takes all the impurities out of your mouth, even all the way up to your sinuses!

Lice Remedy

Begin this all-natural lice treatment with a rinse of apple cider vinegar. Then once the vinegar has dried, apply the oil to your entire head and allow it to sit for twenty-four hours. Brush through your hair with a fine comb and then shampoo again.

Body Lotion

If you're someone who likes to make their own body lotions and other beauty products, then coconut oil is an essential item in your pantry! You can use it to make your own body moisturizer by chilling it, whipping it, and adding a few drops of essential oil. You can also use it plain without whipping or adding the oil for an unscented addition to your routine.

Cuticle Oil

Do you have cracked cuticles in the winter time? Put some coconut oil balm on the base of your nails to remedy that peeling skin and to make your manicure last a little longer!

Brush Cleanser

You should be cleaning your makeup brushes once a month to keep them from getting caked with makeup and building up nasty germs and molds. Use a do it yourself cleanser with two parts antibacterial soap and one part coconut oil. Simply dip the brush in, swirl it around, and then rinse!

Lip Balm

Coconut oil is the best remedy for chapped lips because it's a semisolid at room temperature. Put a little in a miniature jar in the winter time and spread it over your lips during the day with a little brush. You'll have the softest lips around!

Stretch-Mark Cream

Expectant mothers should keep a jar of coconut oil near so that they can ward off those pesky stretch marks, but anyone can use coconut oil as a topical treatment for scars. While the oil doesn't fade marks, it prevents dark spots and blisters from forming.

Under-eye Cream

If you don't want to spend money on expensive under eye creams, use a dab of coconut oil under your eyes and get rid of those bags and fine lines. It's light enough for the delicate skin on your face.

Body Scrub

Mix half a cup of coconut oil with a handful of sugar or coarse salt to make an exfoliator. The moisturizing oil lasts long until the grains have melted away.

Tame Frizzy Hair

Rub a dime sized amount of oil on your hands and them smooth from the midshaft to the ends of your hair for a high-shine finish that gets rid of frizzy hair!

Massage Oil

Warm the coconut oil in the microwave and add a few drops of essential oils, such as peppermint or lavender, for soothing massage oil.

Whitening Toothpaste

Did you run out of toothpaste and you need an alternative? Take your coconut oil and add a little baking soda for a quick fix. Your smile will be really white and healthy!

Shaving Cream

Shaving cream doesn't necessarily have to lather. Take some coconut oil, add a few drops of essential oil, rub it on your legs or face and get started!

Body Oil

Why should you purchase a separate body oil when you keep the coconut oil near the shower? Just slather it on your wet skin after you've showered and pat it dry. You'll be moisturized and you'll also be protected from the sun!

Itch Relief

If you were outside and you got sunburnt, received a few bug bites, or banged your knee on the coffee table again and have a bruise, all of these can be soothed with some coconut oil.

Night Cream

Apply some coconut oil at night for moisturizing benefits all night long. The antioxidants will smooth your fine lines and wrinkles as you sleep.

Deodorant

Mix some coconut oil with a little cornstarch, arrowroot powder, baking soda, and some scented oil for an at-home deodorant!

Coconut oil is a wonderful beauty treatment for both inside and outside the body.

Chapter Five – Using Coconut Oil as an Alternate Treatment for Illnesses and Disease

Coconut oil can be used to treat minor infections all the way up to major illnesses when it's used properly. While it is helpful in treating illnesses and disease, it's always best to be monitored by a doctor while you're being treated.

Fights Inflammation

Coconut oil helps support a healthy endocrine system. According to researchers, coconut oil that is prepared without chemicals or high-heat process has an inhibitory effect on chronic inflammation. Because inflammation is one of the leading causes of most chronic diseases, this study supports that regular consumption of virgin, unprocessed coconut oil helps fight inflammation.

Boosts Immunity

Coconut oil's unique nutrition profile is rich with capric acid, lauric acid, and caprylic acid that provides the body with strong antifungal, antiviral, antibacterial, and antimicrobial properties that have an immune boosting effect. By fighting these factors present in the body, the immune system is better equipped to respond better when it's attacked.

Prevents Bone Loss and Osteoporosis

Oxidative stress and freed radicals are both linked to the development of osteoporosis, which is a metabolic disorder. According to recent research, virgin coconut oil helps maintain bone structure and prevent bone loss in rats that are deficient in estrogen. The study specified virgin coconut oil due to the high polyphenols it has that provide the body with antioxidant properties. The study recommended three tablespoons be taken daily for the best results.

Brain Protector and Alzheimer's Treatment

There are many reports that coconut oil could be a natural treatment for Alzheimer's disease. A current double-blind study recommended taking one tablespoon three times a day to start.

Aids in Sleep

Coconut oil is a great carrier oil when you're making a relaxing and soothing home remedy with essential oils, such as roman chamomile oil or lavender oil. This helps reduce anxiety and helps in getting a good night's rest.

Acne Remedy

Acne is a terrible issue for both adults and teens and is commonly caused by an imbalance of oils in the skin, as well as bacteria overgrowth. Coconut oil is a natural antibiotic and kills the harmful bacteria that lead to the serious outbreak of acne. Try mixing some coconut oil with a little tea tree oil and raw honey for some added effectiveness and benefits.

Cancer Defense and Protection

Medium chain triglycerides and coconut oil have been shown to provide an antitumor effect and they both help provide maintenance for a healthy immune system. This supports the belief that coconut oil helps protect against cancer.

Candida Treatment

Coconut oil has caprylic acid that has an antimicrobial property that aids in killing yeast and candida. In a recent study, researchers discovered that coconut oil was active against many species of candida at a one-hundred percent concentration. It was greater than the drug fluconazole. Add a tablespoon of coconut oil to your diet and apply pure coconut oil to the affected areas twice a day until the symptoms resolve.

Hormone Balancer

The healthy fats found in coconut oil support the adrenal and thyroid glands that lower cortisol and naturally help balance your hormones. Coconut oil aids in suppressing inflammation, while supporting a healthy metabolism, two things that are necessary for balancing hormones. The lauric acid found in coconut oil, as well as many other compounds, supports the adrenal and thyroid glands. This helps lower cortisol in your body to naturally balance the hormones.

Digestive Support

Coconut oil is easy to digest and has compounds that destroy the bad bacteria and promote the growth of good bacteria to help heal leaky gut syndrome. Coconut oil promotes the healthy growth throughout your entire digestive tract. The antifungal, antibacterial, and antimicrobial properties control fungus, parasites, and aid in the efficient utilization of nutrients.

Diabetes Prevention and Blood Glucose Stabilizer

Coconut oil helps to balance your blood glucose levels and has been medically proven to help people with diabetes. It can help balance blood glucose levels by encouraging efficient secretion of insulin from your pancreas. A study conducted in 2009 showed that MCT" are beneficial for preventing obesity and insulin resistance.

Psoriasis and Eczema Treatment

Coconut oil is able to be used as a cream to naturally heal and dry flaking skin for those who have psoriasis and eczema. Mix it with some Shea butter and a little geranium oil for the best effects.

Balance Cholesterol Levels

The healthy fats that are found in coconut oil have been proven to increase the good cholesterol or HDL and bad cholesterol or LDL in the body. According to a study conducted by Harvard Medical School, coconut consumption increased HDL cholesterol and improved the cholesterol ratio.

Constipation Relief

Many people use coconut oil in order to treat prolonged constipation and get rid of their bloating. Try taking a tablespoon at breakfast or at dinner in order to stay regular. The oil penetrates your digestive tract and keeps everything running smoothly by killing off the harmful bacteria and allowing the gut flora to balance itself out.

Heart Disease Treatment

After decades of coconut oil being made to look like a terrible oil due to its saturated fat content, new research has proven that coconut oil is beneficial to heart health because it lowers high blood pressure.

Heals Sick Pets

Just like their human companions, dogs and cats are able to benefit from an addition of coconut oil to their diet. Pets that have digestive upset will benefit from a teaspoon or two added to their food. Skin allergies, wound, and irritations can all be soothed and healed with a topical application of coconut oil. Unlike many other salves, coconut oil is edible and there is no health risk of they lick it off their coat.

Cures UTI's and Kidney Infections

Coconut oil has been used to clear up and heal kidney infections and urinary tract infections. The medium chain fatty acids in the work are a natural antibiotic that disrupts the lipid coating on the bacterium and kill them. In addition, there is a study that showed coconut oil protects the liver from damage. Coconut water also will help keep you hydrated and help the healing process along.

Reduces Symptoms of Pancreatitis and Gallbladder Disease

The medium chain fatty acids of coconut oil don't need the pancreatic enzymes to be broken up, so taking coconut oil eases the strain on your pancreas. In addition, it's so easy to digest that it's been known to improve the symptoms of gallbladder disease, too. Replace other long chain fatty acids with coconut oil to improve your gallbladder and overall body health.

Coconut oil is excellent for health conditions, but it can be used for more than just your body! Learn how to use coconut oil as a cleaner in the next chapter.

Chapter Six – Coconut Oil for the Home

Not only is coconut oil an excellent product for you, but it's also a great way to use something organic and natural to clean your home! This leads to overall much better health because you're not using harsh cleaners around yourself, children, and pets any longer.

Removes Crayon and Gum

Coconut oil is excellent for removing crayon! Just dab some on a cloth and scrub the crayon right off the wall. Follow up with some vinegar to remove any excess oil if your surface is porous.

It also removes gum when it gets stuck in hair, in a carpet, or on the floor. Just rub the spot with oil and allow it to sit for thirty minutes. The oil helps dissolve and loosen the gum.

Prevent Dust

Get out the coconut oil rather than the feather duster next time and coat the high shelves, fans, and other hard to reach areas with oil to prevent dust from building up.

Clean Your Brushes

Dip the soiled hairbrush into a cup of melted coconut oil and wipe the residue off with a towel. Then rinse it with warm after and let it dry before you use it.

Erase Soap Scum

Apply a little coconut oil to a rag and scrub the soap scum right off the side of your tub with ease. Add some baking soda for a little extra scrubbing power if you need to. Avoid flushing it down the drain, though!

Season Cast Iron Skillets

Preheat your oven to 400 degrees Fahrenheit and wipe a thin coating of coconut oil onto every part of the pan. Put the pan on the middle rack of your oven with a cookie sheet beneath it to catch any oil as it melts. Bake it for an hour. To keep the pan properly season, cook with the coconut oil and rub a spoonful on the pan after each washing.

Condition Wood Cutting Boards

Each month, rub some coconut oil on your wooden cutting board to sanitize it and restore it. Leave it for ten minutes and then wipe off the excess oil.

Prevent Rust

Lightly coat the inside of your mason jars with some oil to prevent them from rusting when it's humid out. You can also remove any rust from metal tools by coating it with the coconut oil.

Leave it to rest for an hour and then rinse it with warm water.

Removes Jar Labels

Get rid of the chemical goo removers and use a tablespoon of coconut oil with a tablespoon of baking soda instead! Let it sit for thirty-minute sand then scrape the residue right off. Wash the jar in some hot, soapy water and repeat it when necessary.

Lubricate Hinges

If you have a stiff or a squeaky hinge, just remove the pin in the center and clean and grease it with some coconut oil. Then slide it right back in!

Release Stiff Scissors

Coat the scissor hinge in some coconut oil and leave it for a few minutes. Then wipe the oil off with a soft cloth and the scissors will be easier to use.

Unstick a Zipper

Just use a cotton swab and apply some coconut oil to the zipper's teeth. Try to prevent the oil from getting on the fabric, but if it happens, wash it with a little dish soap.

Clean Guitar Strings

To keep the strings in good shape, dab a clean cloth with some melted coconut oil and then wipe the new strings up and down. Leave them on a clean surface a few minutes, wipe off any excess oil, and then string the guitar. After each session, wipe them with the cloth and clean and lubricate them regularly with the oil.

Coconut oil can be used for just about any household use! Due to its antibacterial, antifungal, and antiviral properties, it can safely clean just about anything.

Chapter Seven – Finding the Right Coconut Oil for Your Needs

There are two different types of coconut oil; those that are mass produced at the industrial level and have to be refined and the ones that begin with fresh coconut and have a shorter refining process. There is no getting around that coconut oil is a naturally refined product because the oil doesn't grow on the tree, the coconuts do. All coconut oil has to be extracted from the whole coconut, so technically speaking, the only true unrefined coconut oil is the one that you consume that's still inside the coconut meat from a fresh coconut that's been picked off the tree.

The term that's used for the least refined coconut oil is virgin coconut oil. Using similar terminology that's used with other edible oils, the term virgin was used with coconut oil in the early twenty-first century to designate the least refined oils that were on the market. The definition of virgin coconut oil was originally created in an internet discussion group and various people had input on the definition. The agreed upon definition is that virgin coconut oil produced without the dried copra as the starting point is virgin.

Copra is the industry-defined term that's used in the Philippines to refer to the dried coconut that has been removed from the shell, but which is inedible and has to be further refined to make the coconut oil. Copra is produced in a few different ways, including sun drying, smoke drying, kiln drying, or derivatives or a combination of any of the aforementioned methods. The one thing that they all have in common is that the product is not suitable for ingestion and has to be further refined. It's smoky, dirty, and it doesn't resemble a food when it comes in the form of copra. Copra is a commodity with its own market price, separate from coconuts, or coconut oil. There are sellers and traders who specifically handle copra in countries that produce coconut oil, and they sell it to coconut oil manufacturing plants. It can be exported to the United States, where it's further processed for manufacturing uses.

So let's look at the different types of refined coconut oil on the market today.

Refined Coconut Oils

In countries where they grow coconuts, these copra-based refined oils are typically mentioned to as RBD coconut oils, which stand for refined, bleach, and deodorized. To bleach the coconut oil, a chemical is not usually used. For this filtering process bleaching clay is used. Steam is used to deodorize the oil because the starting point was copra, which is smoky. So the resulting product has a bland taste with very little or no odor.

One of the misconceptions on the internet is that virgin coconut oil is healthy while refined coconut oil is not, and that refined coconut oils can be harmful. This is usually not true, with a couple of exceptions explained later on. These RBD oils have been on the market for many years now and they are the primary dietary oils that are consumed by billions of people in the tropical climates of the globe. The RBD refining process does not alter the fatty acid profile of the oil, so all the MCT's are kept intact.

What the process does so is strip away from of the nutrients. Virgin coconut oil tests higher in antioxidants. But that doesn't make RBD oils unhealthy.

The types of refined coconut oils you can find on the market today are as follows.

Expeller-Pressed Coconut Oil

This is usually RBD coconut oil produced in a tropical country using a mechanical, physical refining from copra. Physical refining is thought to be cleaner than chemical purifying that utilizes solvent extracts, such as hexane.

Coconut Oil

If there is not a description given and just the plain term of coconut oil is used, then it's most likely an RBD coconut oil. It should be noted that copra is a product that is exported to the United States, where companies refine it for non-edible purposes. Cleaning products and detergents are a common use. With the rise of popularity of coconut oil as edible oil again, some of the large United States manufacturing companies are starting to package coconut oil as edible oil. These cheaper oils are usually mass produced with chemical solvents. While it's unlikely any solvents remain in the finished product, it's still safer to purchase coconut oil for consumption that has not been processed in this way.

Hydrogenated Coconut Oil

This is one of the refined coconut oils that you want to steer clear of as edible oil. The small portion of the unsaturated fatty acids is hydrogenated, which makes a trans-fat. It also keeps the coconut oil solid at a higher temperature. It's unlikely this product is used in the United States, although it could become available in the future. It's better to stay away from this oil. Most coconut oil remains a solid up to seventy-six degree Fahrenheit, and the ambient air temperature is higher in the tropics most of the time. So to keep the coconut oil solid down in the tropics, they hydrogenate it so it can be used in baked goods, candies, and margarine.

Liquid Coconut Oil

This is a new product that appeared available in stores in 2013 and it was called liquid coconut oil that is promoted as coconut oil that stays a liquid despite being put in the refrigerator. It might be a new label, but the product is not new. It's coconut oil that has had the lauric acid removed, so it's fractionated coconut oil. It's also referred to as MCT oil. It's been used in the past in skin care products and more recently as a dietary supplement. It's a refined product that is now marketed as edible oil, but it's actually a by-product of the lauric acid industry. The lauric acid in the coconut oil is known to be the strong antimicrobial component, and it's used as a preservative in many commercial applications. Being a saturated fatty acid, once it's removed, you're left with a liquid that has a much lower melting point. So if you see this product in the store or online, just be aware you are purchasing a highly refined product that is missing one of the most important components, lauric acid.

Virgin Coconut Oil

Now we're going to take a look at virgin coconut oils. As aforementioned, the common denominator that should exist in all virgin oils is that they begin with the fresh coconut and not the copra. However, there is no worldwide certification board that determines or certifies coconut oil as being virgin, so anyone can use the term and put it on the label if they choose to. The first thing to look at when choosing a virgin coconut oil is whether or not it's copra-based or not. If it does use copra as the starting point, then it's not really virgin coconut oil, but industry standard RBD oil that has a nice label.

Extra Virgin Coconut Oil

A common term or title is extra virgin coconut oil. You might be wondering what the difference between extra-virgin and virgin coconut oil is.

It's absolutely nothing. There are no commonly accepted or understood definitions of extra virgin coconut oil like there are in the olive oil industry. It's just a marketing term and nothing else. So when analyzing the virgin coconut oils that are currently available on the market, which would also include those coconut oils that are labeled as being extra virgin, you see that all virgin coconut oils fall into two broad methods of manufacture.

1. Virgin coconut oil that's obtained from pressing the oil out of the dried coconut. With this method, the fresh coconut meat is first dried and then the oil is pressed from the dried coconut. This method is much easier when mass producing virgin coconut oil. The desiccated coconut industry is well established in the countries that produce coconuts, and so these industries have added virgin coconut oil to their production line.
   This is the most common type of virgin or extra virgin oil that you'll find online and in stores. It's mass-produced, but it's still higher quality oil than RBD oil because it begins with fresh and not copra coconut.

2. Virgin coconut oil that's obtained through a wet-milling process. With this method, the oil's extracted from the fresh coconut core without dehydrating the meat first. The coconut milk is expressed by pressing it out of the wet meat. The oil is then further separated from the water. Methods that can be used included fermentation, boiling, enzymes, refrigeration, and mechanical centrifuge.

It's a fortunate thing that coconut oil producing countries did a lot of research on virgin oils over the past decade. They began to wake up to the fact that Western advice on dietary oils, which led to the demonization of the traditional fats and oils such as coconut oil was mostly political in nature rather than scientific.

Most of their research in the recent years has been in the area of heart disease and cholesterol, since this was the main point of attack in the Western countries. They've learned that their traditional oils and fats are in reality better than the expeller-pressed seed oils that come from corn and soy, two crops that are heavily subsided in the United States. This keeps the prices of those oils artificially low.

Researchers from universities in Malaysia, the Philippines, Sri Lanka, and India looked at many different methods of producing coconut oil. At the start, it was hard to determine what could be measured in the laboratory to determine if virgin coconut oil was superior to RBD oil. They soon discovered one characteristic that was able to be measured, and that was significantly higher in virgin oils than RBD oils, which was the level of antioxidants.

Antioxidants are found to be much higher in the virgin coconut oils, especially those that are produced with the wet-milling method.

Process of Wet-Milling

The wet-milling process of creating virgin coconut oil explained above extracts the oil from a wet emulsion or coconut milk. It doesn't press the oil out of the dried coconut. Now, there are many ways to produce coconut oil from wet-milling, and they have different results.

According to many studies, the fermentation wet-milling procedure that uses heat yields the highest levels of antioxidants in virgin coconut oil. The fermentation process is an easier technique of extracting oil, and it's been done in many people's kitchens in the tropical climates for hundreds of years.

During the fermentation process, the milk emulsion is created from freshly grated coconut meat. Then the coconut milk is allowed to sit and ferment for some time, usually overnight. The heavier water sinks to the bottom of the container, leaving the crystal clear layer of oil on top, along with some of the coconut solids. The oil is scooped out into a pan, such as a large wok, and heated for a bit until the solids fall to the bottom of the pan. It's then filtered.

The first research study investigating virgin coconut oil manufacture procedures was released in 2008. This study was done in Malaysia and published in the *International Journal of Food Science Nutrition*. It was the first of its kind reporting that wet-milling fermentation methods produced the highest amounts of antioxidants.

In 2011, research studies were then conducted in Sri Lanka and showed that traditionally wet-milled virgin coconut oil had the highest level of antioxidants. What was surprising was the discovery that the high levels of heat actually increased the amounts of the antioxidants in the oils. This was surprising because there was a misunderstanding stating that heat was detrimental to the coconut oil process, as many virgin oils on the market claimed they were cold pressed or raw and did not use heat.

So virgin coconut oil produced with the wet-milling method that is marked as raw, no heat, or cold pressed actually has fewer antioxidants in it than the heat processed oils.

Therefore, the best type of coconut oil to use is virgin coconut oil that has been processed with heat to extract the most antioxidants.

Conclusion

Coconut oil is an excellent addition to your home; however, it's important you remember that there is such a thing as overuse of a product. While coconut is highly beneficial to you in one to two tablespoon daily doses and can be used on the exterior of your body or for cleaning, it's important not to overconsume coconut oil. It is a laxative and can cause gastric upset if too much is used. To avoid overusing it, it's just best to replace the things you currently use in your home with coconut oil.

In addition, while virgin coconut oil is the best, there is such a thing as organic coconut oil. Organic coconut oil is often virgin coconut oil, but be sure it's processed with heat if you want to get the most benefits out of it. Remember, cold-processed and raw coconut oil have a lower amount of antioxidants than heat processed oils.

I hope you enjoyed this book about coconut oil and its uses and benefits. If you did, please leave a review on Amazon. Every review counts!

Thank you for reading.

BEFORE YOU GO

Free Gift

As Promised Here Is Your Guide To
Spiritual Techniques To Heal Your Body
And Soul

Get Your Copy Now

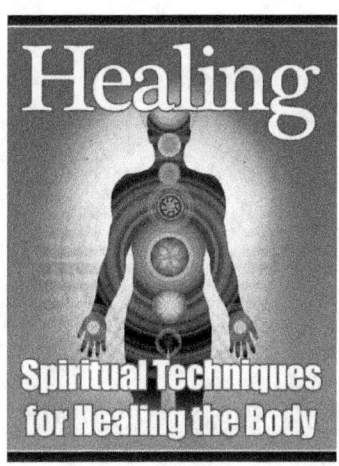

LEARN HOW TO GET MORE DONE IN A DAY

Do you feel stuck and stressed because of the constant damage on your body and mind, both physically and spiritually? Or do you know someone that is hurt beyond than just the soul? Spiritual healing is the ability of your mind and soul to repair your ailments. These ailments are not limited mere physical wounds, but can also relate to mental illness and self esteem issues. Many modern day physicians invoke the idea of spiritual healing along with western medicine as a means to promote the health of their patients. This can dramatically change your life physically and spiritually. Take action now!

Download Healing To Change Your Life!

If You Want Free Best Selling Kindle Books Delivered Straight To Your Inbox

JOIN OUR FREE KINDLE BOOK CLUB!

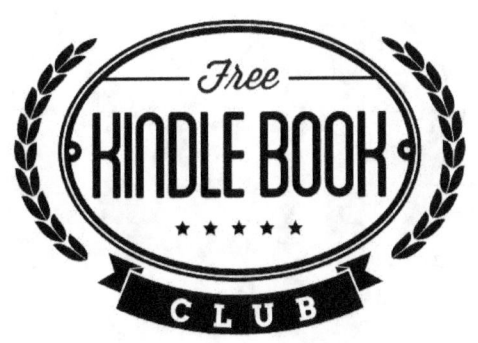

CLICK HERE

Thank you again for downloading this book!

If you enjoyed this book, then I'd like to ask you for a favor, would you be kind enough to leave a review for this book on Amazon? It'd be greatly appreciated!

Thank you and good luck! ☺

Tiffany Thorton

www.ingramcontent.com/pod-product-compliance
Lightning Source LLC
Chambersburg PA
CBHW071134280526
45787CB00003B/1285